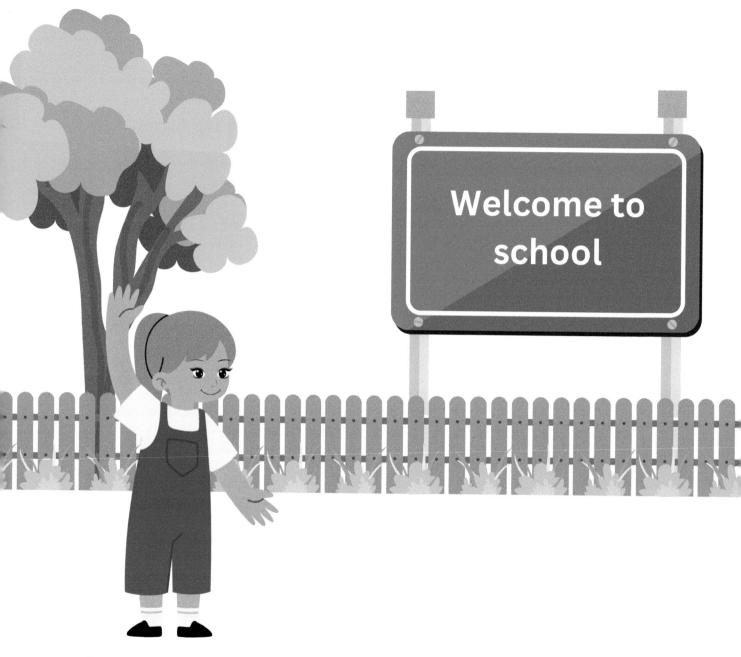

Hi there! My name is Gwen. I love doing fun things like reading, dancing, and playing with my friends.

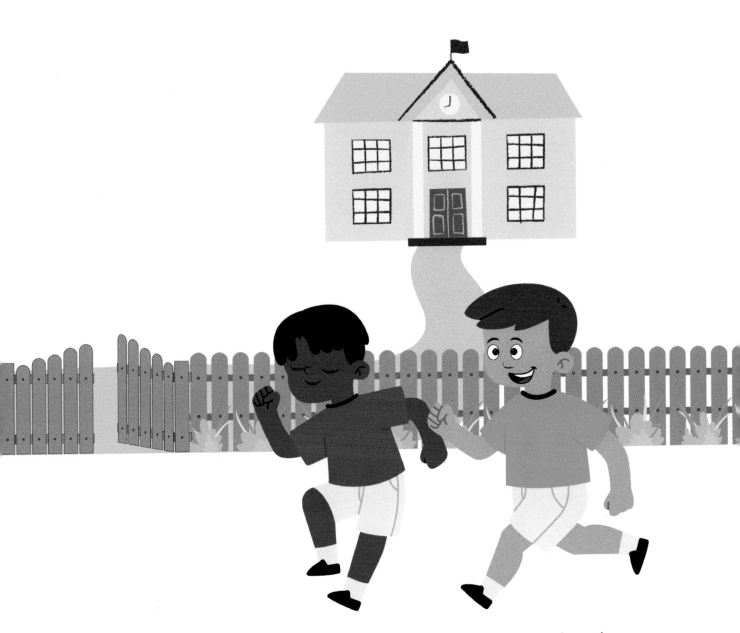

I have lots of friends, and two of them, Amir and Toby, are just like me - they're autistic too!

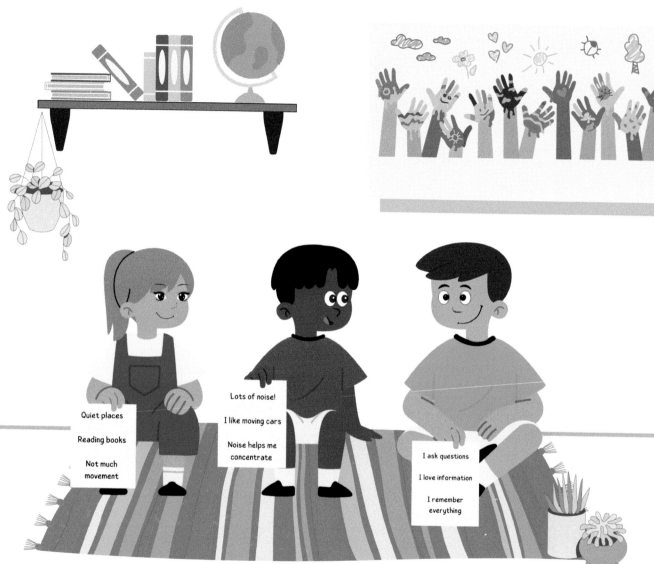

Being autistic means that our brains work a little differently to most people's brains. Even though we're all autistic, our brains like different things. You see, our brains are like recipes, and they need different ingredients to work well.

Amir's brain likes noisy and busy places. He enjoys watching traffic on busy roads because it helps his brain work better. When Amir needs to concentrate, he likes to have lots of noise around him.

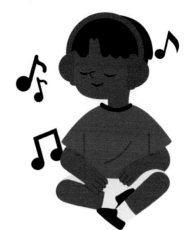

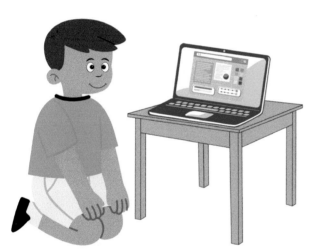

Toby's brain loves information. It's like a super smart computer that remembers everything he learns.

My brain prefers a peaceful and quiet place with not too much going on. I like to learn by reading books quietly.

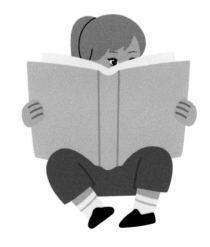

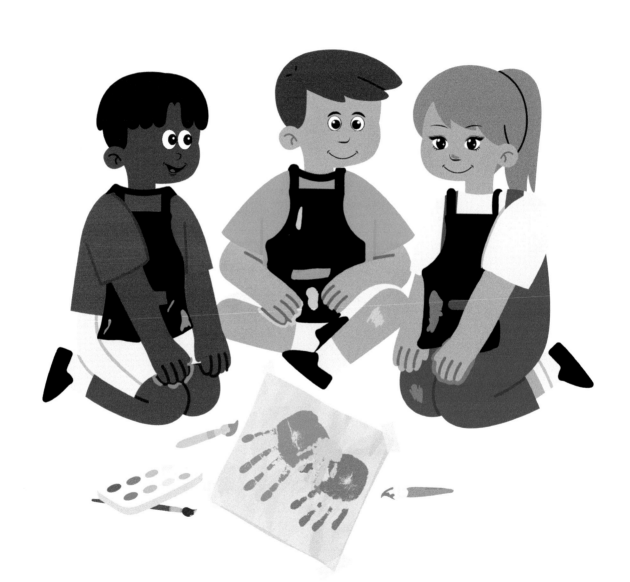

Even though our brains are different, there are some things that all autistic brains have in common. We experience life in a unique way compared to most people.

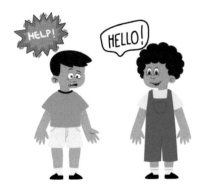

Sometimes, it's hard for us to communicate or understand what others are saying.

We also process information from our senses (like what we see, hear, touch, and smell) differently.

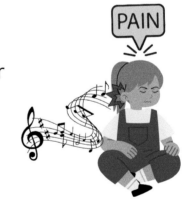

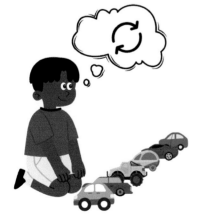

And we like things to be done in a similar way, so we enjoy repetition.

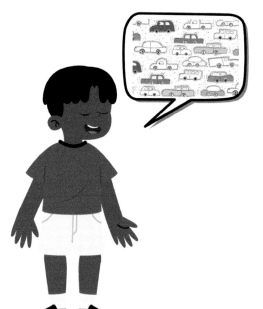

Communication can be tricky for autistic people. We all have different ways of talking and expressing ourselves. Amir loves to talk about cars a lot, while Toby finds it hard to look at people when he talks to them.

He asks a lot of questions but doesn't like it when someone asks him about his feelings. Sometimes Toby uses a tablet to communicate instead of talking.

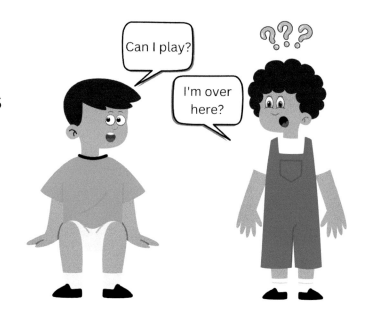

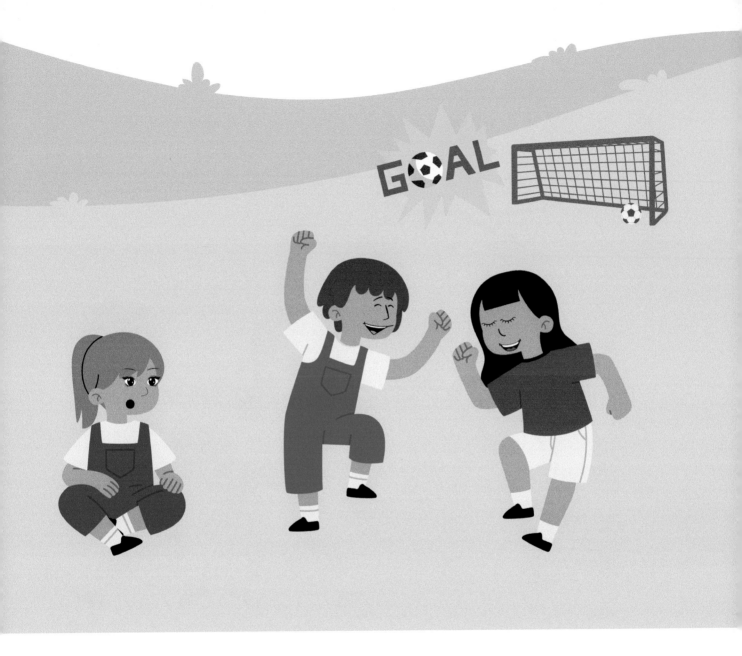

As for me, I sometimes struggle with knowing what to say or how to behave, so I look at other people and copy them.

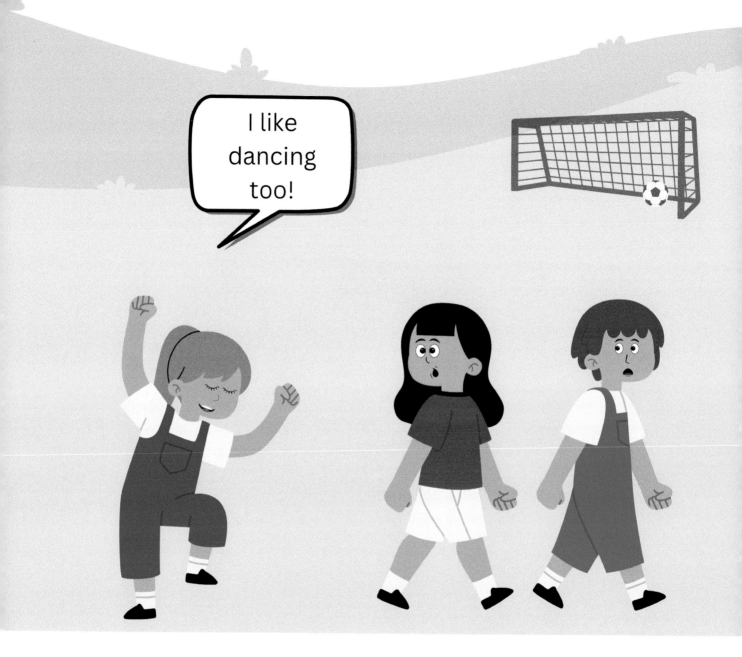

But that means I might say or do the wrong things sometimes.

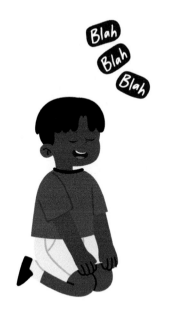

Autistic people communicate in many different ways. Some use talking, sign language, or writing and drawings. Some even use special devices like iPads or computers.

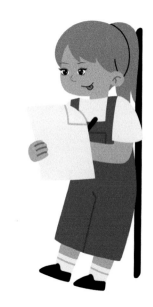

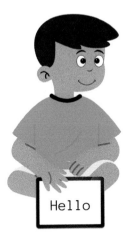

No matter how we communicate, there are certain things we might feel or ways we might react.

For example, we might find it hard to understand what others are saying, or listen in noisy places. Sometimes we might even become nonverbal and unable to speak, even if we normally can.

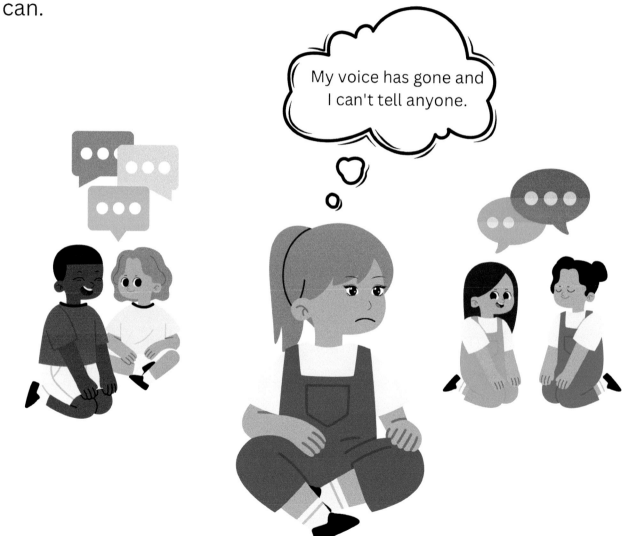

Our brains also help us process information from our senses. That means how we see, hear, touch, and smell things.

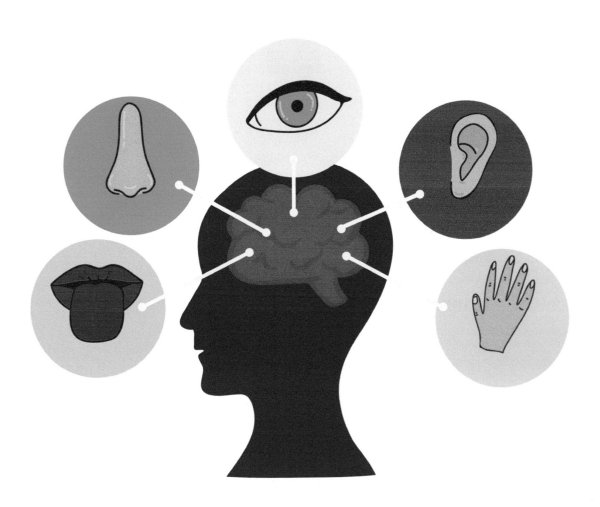

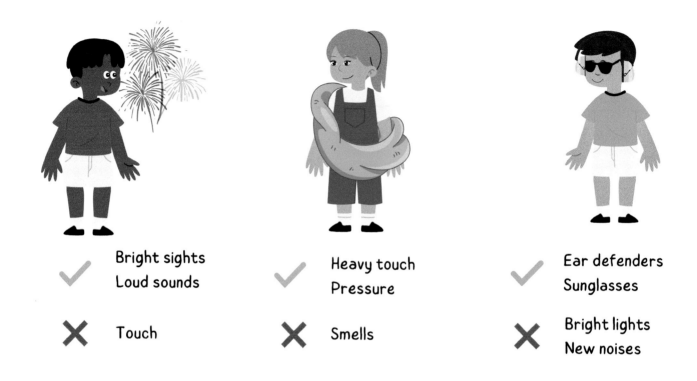

✓	Bright sights Loud sounds
✗	Touch

✓	Heavy touch Pressure
✗	Smells

✓	Ear defenders Sunglasses
✗	Bright lights New noises

Amir's brain works best with lots of sounds and sights around him, but he doesn't like being touched too much.

Toby gets scared by unfamiliar noises and bright lights, so he wears ear defenders and sunglasses to help him.

I don't like certain smells because they make my brain feel overwhelmed. But I find calmness and relaxation when I have pressure, like using a heavy blanket.

Autistic people like routine and don't like sudden changes. It can be hard for our brains to process new things. We use different ways to help us prepare for the day ahead.

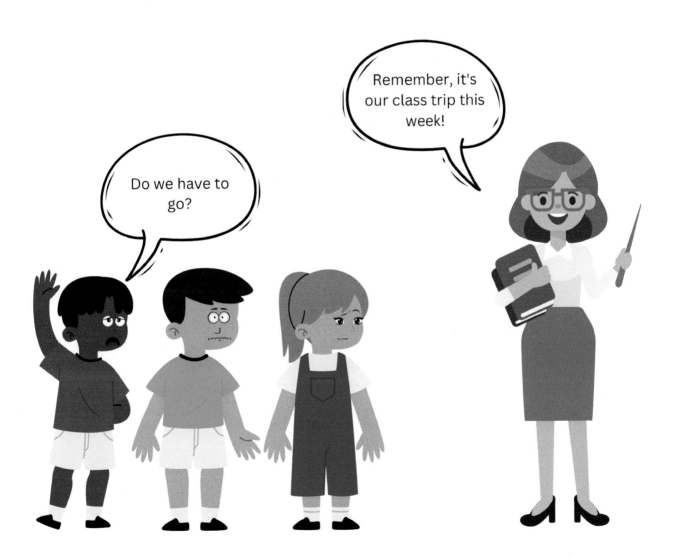

For example, Amir uses a timetable to know what's coming next.

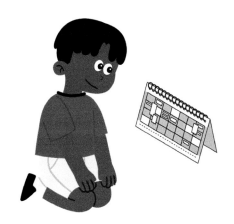

Toby likes to repeat things many times to remember them,

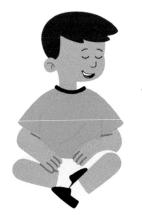

"We are going on a school trip."

"We are going on a school trip."

"We are going on a school trip."

and I prefer to focus on what I'm doing right now and what comes next with the help of cards.

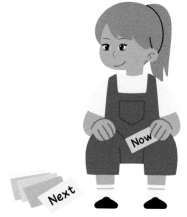

Sometimes our brains can become overwhelmed or overloaded. This can happen in different ways. It's like a bottle of fizzy drink that gets shaken too much and then explodes when opened. We call it a meltdown.

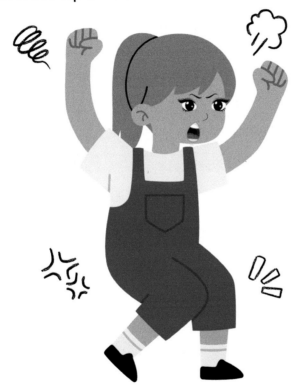

During a meltdown, autistic people might cry, shout, hit, kick, or throw things. But it's important to remember that we're not being naughty. We're just not in control of our brains at that moment.

Sometimes when someone feels really overwhelmed or has too much going on, they can get tired or go very quiet.

It can be just like a deflated beach ball. Imagine you have a beach ball that gets stuck on shells and rocks on the beach. You try to blow it back up, but it keeps getting more and more holes in it until there's no air left. Then the ball becomes flat and you can't play with it anymore.

When an autistic person has run out of energy, sometimes they can't play or talk. This is called a shutdown.

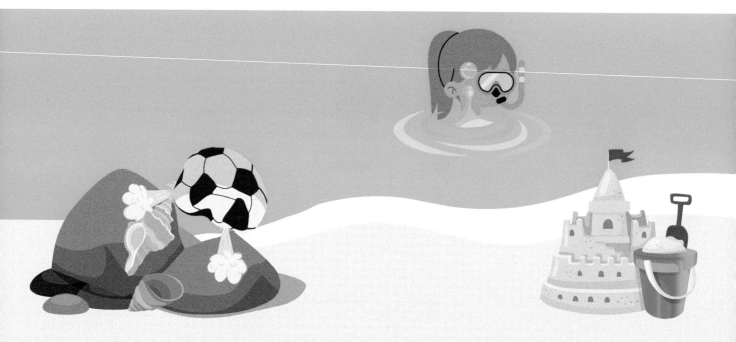

Shutdowns can look different for each autistic person. Some might fall asleep even if they're in the middle of a class at school.

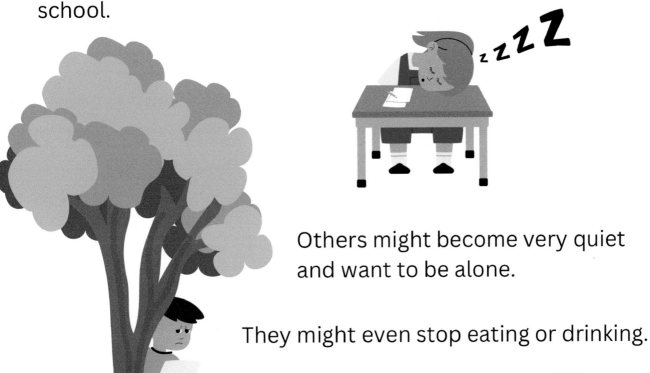

Others might become very quiet and want to be alone.

They might even stop eating or drinking.

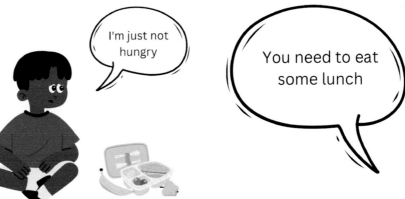

I'm just not hungry

You need to eat some lunch

Sometimes meltdowns and shutdowns don't happen right away when someone feels overwhelmed. It's like keeping a lid on a bottle or the beach ball staying inflated until the person is in a safe place.

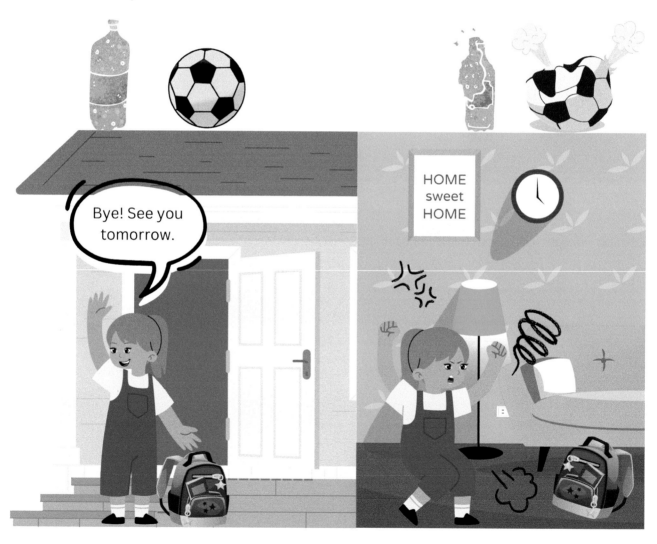

When an autistic person is masking, it means they're trying to hide their autism. Not everyone does this, but some people, like Amir and me, do.

When Amir masks, he might say "yes" to things even if he wants to say something else, just to make things easier.

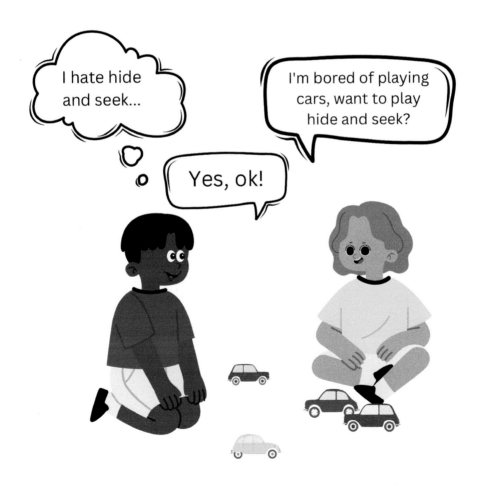

I mask when I'm in a new situation and don't know what to do. I watch other people to figure out how to act.

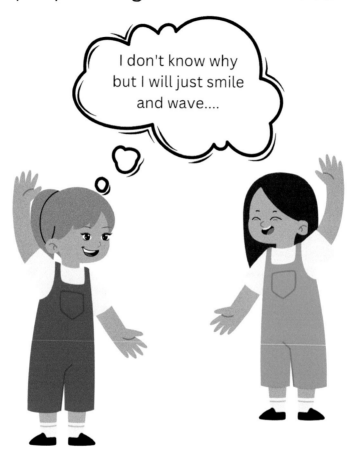

Masking can be tiring, but it doesn't mean we're ashamed of being autistic. Sometimes it's just easier for us, even if it makes us tired later on.

Eating can be difficult for autistic people too. Amir likes certain foods, but he has specific ways he wants them served, like in bowls with his favorite cartoon characters. Toby prefers beige-coloured foods like potatoes, chicken, and rice. I eat more colourful food, but I can't have different foods touching on my plate. It helps me focus on one taste and texture at a time. When we go to other people's houses for dinner, we might bring our own food or let them know about what we need.

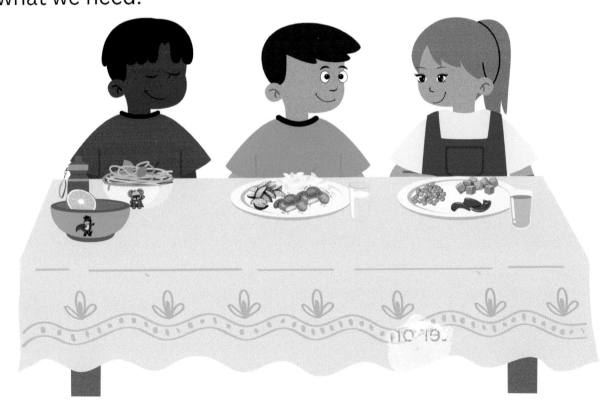

Stimming is something everyone does to feel good, like tapping your fingers on a table. Autistic people stim more because it helps us calm down and express our feelings.

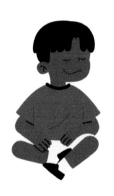 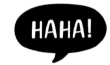

Amir hums, claps, and laughs when he's happy.

Toby flaps his hands and spins around.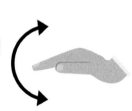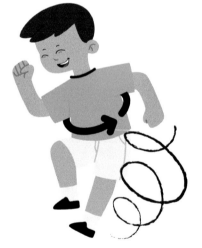

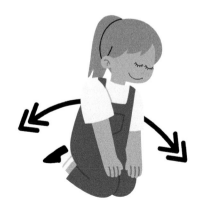 I rock back and forth to feel calm.

We all learn in different ways because our autism affects us differently. Amir found it hard to understand lessons at our local school. Now he goes to a school with fewer children and more adults to help him follow instructions.

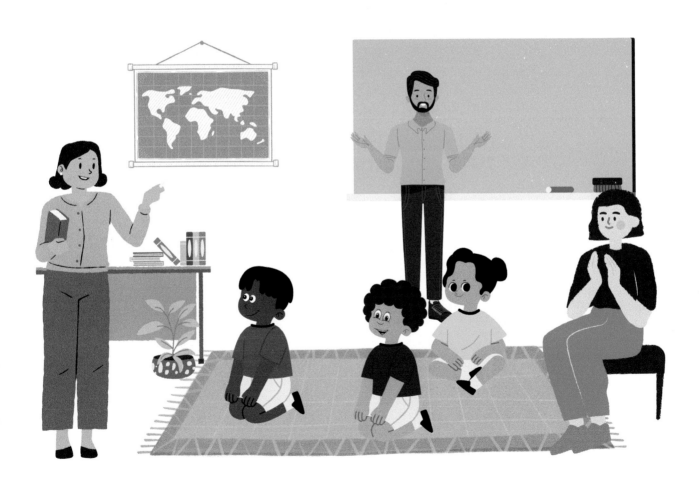

After trying our local school, Toby now learns at home. He loves learning new things and being outdoors.

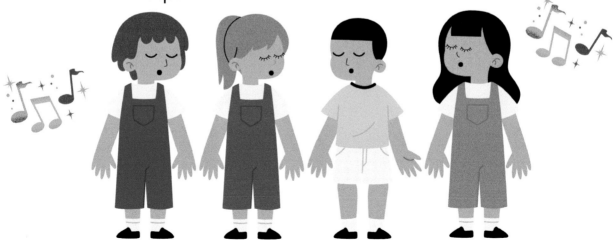

I go to the school near my house and sometimes need a little support, but I can do most things just like other kids. My friends who are not autistic are really kind and helpful when I need a little help.

Having friends makes me happy, even though it can be hard to understand the rules of games sometimes. When I play with Amir, he likes his cars and wants me to play nearby without touching them. When I play with Toby, we do science experiments together.

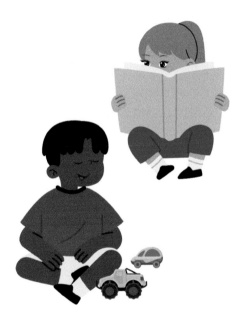

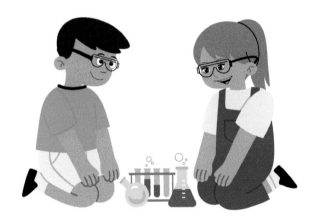

Going to places like the cinema with friends who aren't autistic is fun for me too, because I can enjoy their company without having to talk too much.

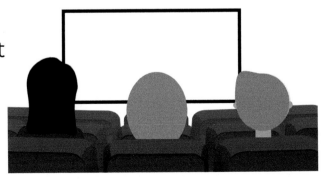

Being autistic is nothing to worry about. It can be awesome, and there are many famous autistic people who have done important things.

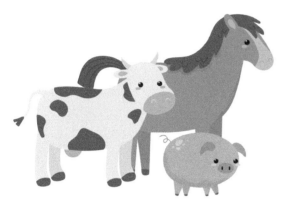

Temple Grandin has made changes in how farm animals are cared for,

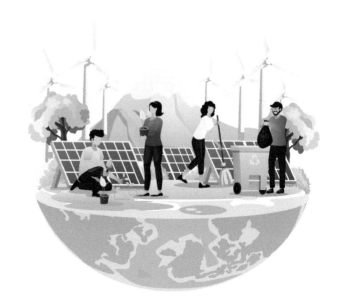

and Greta Thunberg is an environmentalist making a big impact on helping us all to care for our planet.

Every autistic person has their own abilities. They can be....

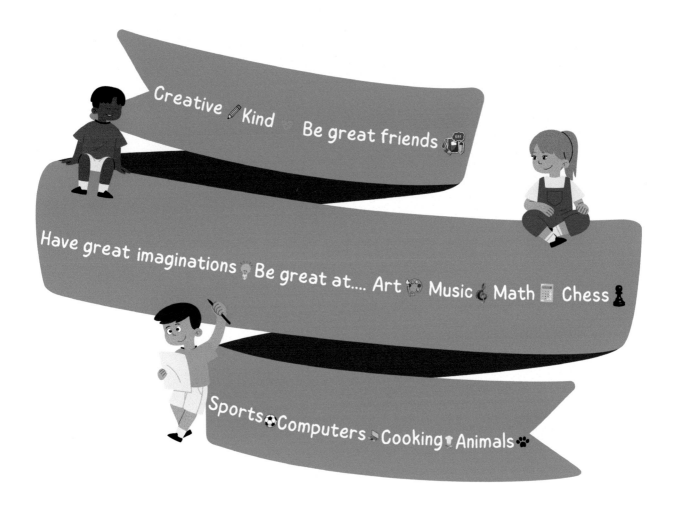

Creative ✏️ Kind 🌸 Be great friends 🎒

Have great imaginations 💡 Be great at.... Art 🎨 Music 🎵 Math 🧮 Chess ♟️

Sports ⚽ Computers 🖱️ Cooking 🍴 Animals 🐾

The list goes on and on, and being autistic is something to be proud of.

For educational resources to use with this book, visit our website www.autability.co.uk